The 40-Count Plan
Forty Days and Forty Counts to Wellness

PINKIE A. HOLMES

AND

DEBRA LA CHELLE DUPREE

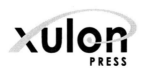

Copyright © 2011 by Pinkie A. Holmes

The 40-Count Plan
Forty Days and Forty Counts to Wellness
by Pinkie A. Holmes and Debra La Chelle Dupree

Printed in the United States of America

ISBN 9781600344732

All rights reserved solely by the author. The author guarantees all contents are original and do not infringe upon the legal rights of any other person or work. No part of this book may be reproduced in any form without the permission of the author. The views expressed in this book are not necessarily those of the publisher.

Scripture quotations marked (AMP) are taken from The Amplified® Bible, Copyright © 1954, 1958, 1962, 1964, 1965, 1987 by The Lockman Foundation. Used by permission. (www.Lockman.org)

Scripture quotations marked (The Message) are taken from The Message. Copyright © 1993, 1994, 1995, 1996, 2000, 2001, 2002. Used by permission of NavPress Publishing Group.

NOTE: *Pronouns referring to God, Jesus, and the Holy Spirit have been capitalized in all Scripture verses.*

Cover Concept by Pinkie A. Holmes, Debra La Chelle Dupree and Xulon Press

Design by Xulon Press

www.xulonpress.com

Dedication

To my mother, Pinkie M. Whetstone

and

To all those who are able to include physical exercise in their everyday lives but keep making excuses for not exercising and to those people who may be physically challenged, confined to the bed, or need a less strenuous exercise program. You can do all things through Christ, Who strengthens you to do the things that He wants you to do. He certainly wants you to be healthy. All you need is the will to try. You will be the victor and get to the finish line forty days and forty counts at a time.

"Nothing beats failure but a try." –Pinkie M. Whetstone

Disclaimer

If you have any medical conditions, including but not limited to heart disease, diabetes, or a family history of illness, please speak with a medical practitioner before starting any exercise or diet plan.

The authors of this book are not nor do they claim to be certified exercise trainers or health professionals. They simply did these exercises, followed the diet plans, and are on their way to a more physically, mentally, and spiritually healthier way of living.

Contents

Disclaimer vii
Acknowledgments xiii
Introduction xvii
Breathing In and Out xxi

CHAPTER ONE
    Day 1: Face Stretch 25
    Day 2: The Stand 27
    Day 3: Knee Bend 29
    Day 4: Hand Tightening 31
    Day 5: Open Wide 33
    Day 6: With Open Arms 35
    Day 7: Hugging Yourself 37

    DIET PLANS FOR THE 40-COUNT PLAN
        Option 1: Self-Control-Rooted Diet Plan 39
        Option 2: Discipline-Rooted Diet Plan 40
        Option 3: Self-Control/Discipline-Rooted
            Diet Plan 41

    GOD'S PLAN: For Total Renewal (Including
        Prayer of Salvation) 42

Day 8: Body Twists 45

CHAPTER TWO
Day 9: Leg Raise 49
Day 10: Leg Hugs 51
Day 11: Happy Shoulders 53
Day 12: Tummy Tuck 55
Day 13: Head Moves 57
Day 14: One-Legged Stand 59
Day 15: Flat-out Stretching 61
Day 16: Toe Stretch 63

CHAPTER THREE
Day 17: Elbow Stretch 67
Day 18: Almost Sitting 69
Day 19: Stretch and Lift 71
Day 20: Moving Still 73
Day 21: Swimming on Dry Land 75
Day 22: Uplifting Praise 77
Day 23: Thigh Togetherness 79
Day 24: Arm Lift 81

CHAPTER FOUR
Day 25: Body Stretching 85
Day 26: Eye Strengthening 87
Day 27: Thigh Massage 89
Day 28: Piano Move 91
Day 29: Graceful Arms 93
Day 30: Leg Strengthening 95
Day 31: Heel/Toe 97
Day 32: Nostril Opening 99

CHAPTER FIVE
Day 33: Drawing a Moon 103
Day 34: Upper Body Stretch 105

Day 35: Bend, Slide, Squat 107
Day 36: Side Kick 109
Day 37: Bowing Down 111
Day 38: Standing Firm 113
Day 39: Shake It Off 115
Day 40: Defining Muscle 117

Conclusion 119
Appendix 123

Acknowledgments

With special thanks to:

Sherman Holmes, for your love and support.

Ruth Teal, Mary Moton, Richard Whetstone, Valeria Thornton, and Charles Whetstone, for your love.

Debra La Chelle Dupree, for your hard work, dedication, and belief in my vision for this book.

Sophie Dawn Braxton, for your counsel and proofreading expertise.

Jeanette A. Cameron of Risen Editing, for your excellent editing work in helping to produce a masterpiece.

The Xulon Press Team, for your guidance, creativity, work, and support in the production of the book.

Beloved, I pray that you may prosper in every way and [that your body] may keep well, even as [I know] your soul keeps well and prospers. (3 John 1:2 AMP)

Introduction

This is a daily devotional and motivational wellness book designed for your total renewal. The path to physical, mental, and spiritual well-being outlined in this book is a way of life—a unique approach to wellness. The regimen includes forty days of prayer, Scripture, and counts (repetitions) of physical exercise. Included are unique diet plans designed to root you in self-control and discipline and a plan that will renew your mind and enter you into an extraordinary life. I do not believe that overeating is the only reason why most people are overweight. I think that lack of self-control and discipline are at the root of the problem. I hope that you take complete advantage of all that this book has to offer since it was created to help you develop the tools to defeat temptation of all kinds, promote good habits, and give you extraordinary results. If you follow the forty-day plan to its fullest, the possibilities are endless.

In the biblical events listed below, God used forty days to bring something to pass as well as to create something new, mostly life in some form. After it rained on the earth for forty days and forty nights, the earth was wiped clean and new living substances and things were created. Moses spent forty days and forty nights with God, without eating bread or drinking water, and was given the Ten Commandments, which established laws for the Israelites. The Scriptures below mention these events and others that took place in a forty-day time period:

> For in seven days I will cause it to rain upon the earth forty days and forty nights, and every living substance and thing that I have made I will destroy, blot out, and wipe away from the face of the earth. (Genesis 7:4 AMP)

> So he arose and ate and drank, and went in the strength of that food forty days and nights to Horeb, the mount of God. (1 Kings 19:8 AMP)

> To them also He showed Himself alive after His passion (His suffering in the garden and on the cross) by [a series of] many convincing demonstrations [unquestionable evidences and infallible proofs], appearing to them during forty days and talking [to them] about the things of the kingdom of God. (Acts 1:3 AMP)

> Moses was there with the Lord forty days and forty nights; he ate no bread and drank no water. And he wrote upon the tables the words of the covenant, the Ten Commandments. (Exodus 34:28 AMP)

> And they returned from scouting out the land after forty days. (Numbers 13:25 AMP)

> The Philistine came out morning and evening, presenting himself for forty days. (1 Samuel 17:16 AMP)

The 40-Count Plan

THEN JESUS was led (guided) by the [Holy] Spirit into the wilderness (desert) to be tempted (tested and tried) by the devil. And He went without food for forty days and forty nights, and later He was hungry. And the tempter came and said to Him, If You are God's Son, command these stones to be made [loaves of] bread. But He replied, It has been written, Man shall not live and be upheld and sustained by bread alone, but by every word that comes forth from the mouth of God. (Matthew 4:1-4 AMP)

If God chose forty days for these biblical events, I feel that forty days is sufficient to create a healthier body, soul, and spirit. Once you have completed the initial forty days of exercises, the diet plans, and the total renewal plan, I hope you will repeat the exercises and continue the plans. One suggestion would be to create a personal, daily wellness regimen and incorporate all of your favorite exercises from the book. The key is to make wellness a normal part of your life. *The 40-Count Plan* is about you, with God's help, developing healthier habits in your daily routine and creating a physically mentally, and spiritually healthier you.

ICON NOTE: *All exercises that can be performed in bed will be indicated with this icon.*

Breathing In and Out

Before we get started, it is important that you learn the breathing technique for each exercise.

Take a deep breath in through your nose and then release slowly, breathing out through your nose. It is said that you should inhale on the easiest movement and exhale on the hardest. If you decide to breathe this way, this would mean that you begin by releasing slowly, breathing out through your nose, and then taking a deep breath in through your nose, instead of the reverse. I believe that whichever way you choose is fine, as long as you remember to breathe. It is equally important to maintain a comfortable pace of breathing throughout your routine. The most important thing is not to overwork your heart and have it enter a danger zone. That would defeat the purpose of the book.

Let's get started!

CHAPTER ONE

Day 1

Warm-Up Prayer:

Let us begin by bowing, or lifting, our heads to pray. You can pray silently or aloud, as long as it is heartfelt prayer. For those of you who do not know how to pray, just speak with your hearts to God about the exercises you are about to attempt and the results you'd like to achieve.

Dear Father, please guide me into doing each exercise just as it should be done and let me reap the benefits that it will bring me. Please help me to eat right and, in forty days, be healthier physically, mentally, and spiritually. In Jesus' Name, Amen.

Exercise: Face Stretch

Always remember to breathe in and out through your nose. Push your lips out in a pouting position and move your lips and cheeks from left to right. Repeat this for twenty counts. Move the upper half of your face up by raising your eyebrows upwards as high as possible then release. Repeat this for ten counts and then move the bottom part of your face, stretching your facial muscles downwards towards your neck for ten counts. To see what muscles you are working, you can do this exercise while looking in the mirror.

NOTE: This exercise can be performed in a standing, sitting, or lying position. The goal is always to try to do a total of forty counts of the exercises. Because some of us are at different exercising levels, including never having exercised before, it may seem difficult at first. However, if you do as much as you are capable of doing, I promise that by the time you reach Day 40, you will rejoice in your diligence.

Cool-Down Scripture (Speak This):

Lean on, trust in, and be confident in the Lord with all your heart and mind and do not rely on your own insight or understanding. In all your ways know, recognize, and acknowledge Him, and He will direct and make straight and plain your paths. (Proverbs 3:5-6 AMP)

Day 2

Warm-Up Prayer:

Let us begin by bowing, or lifting, our heads and praying a heartfelt prayer. Speak with your hearts to God about the exercises you are about to attempt and the results you'd like to achieve. Your prayer could be the same or something different from Day 1. Normally, any time after I have prayed for something that I know is in God's Will, I give thanks to the Lord.

Dear Father, thank You for guiding me into doing each exercise just as it should be done and letting me reap the health benefits that it will bring me. Thank You for helping me to eat right and, in forty days, be healthier physically, mentally, and spiritually. In Jesus' Name, Amen.

Exercise: The Stand

Always remember to breathe in and out through your nose. Stand with your hands placed on your waist or hips, whichever is more comfortable, and hold that position for a minute. Stretch your arms out to the sides and move them in a circular motion frontwards, repeating for five counts and backwards for five counts. Place your hands back on your waist or hips, whichever is more comfortable, and hold that position for a minute. Take your right leg and bring it frontwards, raising it as high as you can, and bring it back down to the floor. Take your right leg and bring it towards the back, raising it as high as you can, and bring it back down to the floor. Repeat this for ten counts. Then do the left side. Remember to relax as needed.

NOTE: This exercise should be performed in a standing position only.

Cool-Down Scripture (Speak This):

I have strength for all things in Christ Who empowers me [I am ready for anything and equal to anything through Him Who infuses inner strength into me; I am self-sufficient in Christ's sufficiency]. (Philippians 4:13 AMP)

Day 3

Warm-Up Prayer:

Let us bow, or lift, our heads and pray. You can pray your own prayer, use the one below, or do both.

Dear Father, thank You for continuing to guide me into doing each exercise just as it should be done and continuing to let me reap the health benefits that it will bring me. Thank You for continuing to help me to eat right and, in forty days, be healthier physically, mentally, and spiritually. In Jesus' Name, Amen.

Exercise: Knee Bend

Always remember to breathe in and out through your nose. Lie down on your back and place your hands behind your head in a locking position. Bring your knees in towards your chest and then slowly stretch your legs back out, keeping the feet from touching the floor. Repeat this exercise for forty counts. Remember to rest as needed.

NOTE: *This exercise should be performed in a lying position only and may be more easily done with a pillow placed under your backside (buttocks).*

Cool-Down Scripture (Speak This):

Love never gives up. Love cares more for others than for self. Love doesn't want what it doesn't have. Love doesn't strut, Doesn't have a swelled head, Doesn't force itself on others, Isn't always "me first," Doesn't fly off the handle, Doesn't keep score of the sins of others, Doesn't revel when others grovel, Takes pleasure in the flowering of truth, Puts up with anything, Trusts God always, Always looks for the best, Never looks back, But keeps going to the end. (1 Corinthians 13:4-7 The Message)

Day 4

Warm-Up Prayer:

Let us bow, or lift, our heads and pray. You can pray your own prayer, use the one below, or do both.

Dear Father, thank You for blessing me with Your wisdom and discernment. I wholeheartedly respect You and turn away from that which is evil. Thank You for excellent health in my body and nourishment in my bones. In Jesus' Name, Amen.

Exercise: Hand Tightening

Always remember to breathe in and out through your nose. Place your arms out in front of you, bring both hands together and push with your arms into your hands where your hands and palms touch tightly. Hold this for a count of forty. For less pressure, push lightly and bring your arms more in towards your chest.

NOTE: *This exercise can be performed in a standing, sitting, or lying position. Remember to rest as needed.*

Cool-Down Scripture (Speak This):

Don't assume that you know it all. Run to God! Run from evil! Your body will glow with health, your very bones will vibrate with life! (Proverbs 3:7-8 The Message)

Day 5

Warm-Up Prayer:

Let us bow, or lift, our heads and pray. You can pray your own prayer, use the Scripture prayer below, or do both.

Pray, therefore, like this: Our Father Who is in Heaven, hallowed (kept holy) be Your name. Your kingdom come, Your will be done on earth as it is in Heaven. Give us this day our daily bread. And forgive us our debts, as we also have forgiven (left, remitted, and let go of the debts, and have given up resentment against) our debtors. And lead (bring) us not into temptation, but deliver us from the evil one. For Yours is the kingdom and the power and the glory forever. Amen. (Matthew 6:9-13 AMP)

Exercise: Open Wide

Always remember to breathe in and out through your nose. Open your mouth as wide as possible, forming the shape of an "O." Really stretch your mouth muscles as much as possible. Smile the largest smile possible, bringing teeth together to the point of feeling the stretch in your cheek muscles. Repeat this exercise for forty counts. Rest as needed.

NOTE: This exercise can be performed in a standing, sitting, or lying position.

Cool-Down Scripture (Speak This):

There's an opportune time to do things, a right time for everything on the earth: A right time for birth and another for death, A right time to plant and another to reap, A right time to kill and another to heal, A right time to destroy and another to construct, A right time to cry and another to laugh, A right time to lament and another to cheer, A right time to make love and another to abstain, A right time to embrace and another to part, A right time to search and another to count your losses, A right time to hold on and another to let go, A right time to rip out and another to mend, A right time to shut up and another to speak up, A right time to love and another to hate, A right time to wage war and another to make peace. (Ecclesiastes 3:1-8 The Message)

Day 6

Warm-Up Prayer:

Let us bow, or lift, our heads and pray. You can pray your own prayer, use the one below, or do both.

And forgive us our debts, as we also have forgiven (left, remitted, and let go of the debts, and have given up resentment against) our debtors. (Matthew 6:12 AMP)

Dear Father, please help me to acknowledge the mercy that is Yours, the same mercy that You have equipped me with. Please help me to truly forgive in the way in which You have modeled so that I too can be forgiven by my Heavenly Father in the same way. In Jesus' Name, Amen.

Exercise: With Open Arms

Always remember to breathe in and out through your nose. Stretch both arms out to the sides and make fists. Bring both arms to the front of you where both fists touch. Keep your hands as fists and stretch both arms back out to the side and lower back down. Repeat for forty counts. Rest as needed.

NOTE: This exercise can be performed in a standing, sitting, or lying position.

Cool-Down Scripture (Speak This):

Pray, therefore, like this: Our Father Who is in Heaven, hallowed (kept holy) be Your name. Your kingdom come, Your will be done on earth as it is in Heaven. Give us this day our daily bread. And forgive us our debts, as we also have forgiven (left, remitted, and let go of the debts, and have given up resentment against) our debtors. And lead (bring) us not into temptation, but deliver us from the evil one. For Yours is the kingdom and the power and the glory forever. Amen. (Matthew 6:9-13 AMP)

NOTE: The above Scripture has been repeated intentionally. This Scripture has great benefits. It is the example of how Jesus instructs us to pray, and most of us just say it without fully paying attention to the words.

Day 7

Warm-Up Prayer:

Let us bow, or lift, our heads and pray. You can pray your own prayer, use the one below, or do both.

Dear Father, I praise Your Holy Name. Your mercy and loving-kindness are great towards me. Your truth and faithfulness endure forever. In Jesus' Name, Amen.

Exercise: Hugging Yourself

Always remember to breathe in and out through your nose. Hold out your arms and hug yourself, with your right hand touching your left shoulder, with all of your might. Bring your arms back out and hug yourself again, but this time with your left hand touching your right shoulder. Do this for forty counts, alternating sides each time. Rest as needed.

NOTE: *This exercise can be performed in a standing, sitting, or lying position.*

Cool-Down Scripture (Speak This):

When God approves of your life, even your enemies will end up shaking your hand. (Proverbs 16:7 The Message)

DIET PLANS FOR THE 40-COUNT PLAN

You may choose to follow one, two, or all three of the following diet plans during each 40-day cycle.

Option 1:
Self-Control-Rooted Diet Plan
(Begin on Day 8 or Day 15)

Like the exercise regimen, the diet plans in this book are designed to give you excellent mental and physical health. With this in mind, they will not follow typical diet plans that limit you to a certain amount of vegetables, fat, protein, fruits, carbohydrates, and dairy. Instead, I am suggesting that you give up the most enjoyable, fattening treat that you eat on a regular basis. It is said that 3500 calories burned equal one pound lost.

I took a look at what it would be like if I gave up eating ice cream. Let's say I eat a little over a cup (a nice serving at 8.5 oz) of butter-pecan ice cream once a week. Each serving contains 705 calories. 705 calories x 52 weeks = 36,660 calories. Dividing 36,660 by 3500 calories = more than 10 pounds (actual 10.47). By just giving up the serving of ice cream that I have once a week, I should lose approximately 10 pounds in one year's time. This also means that if I continue to eat my ice cream, I will have to double the calories burned (burn off the ice cream calories and an additional 705 calories) in order to see the 10-pound weight loss at the end of the year. However, if I give up the ice cream *in addition to* burning 705 calories per week I should lose approximately 20 pounds by the end of the year.

If I give up the ice cream for only forty days, I should lose about one pound. I used ice cream as an example. You may want to give up that cookie, package of cookies, or bag of chips you like so much. Maybe even the fattening cream that you put in your coffee. You be the judge of what you should give up for the next forty days. But I want you to give up something. In the process, it will teach you self-control.

Option 2:
Discipline-Rooted Diet Plan
(Begin on Day 8 or Day 15)

This diet is designed to help you gain discipline in never letting food control you again. Through this diet, you will become more disciplined, and the gratification received will be a welcome emotion that you will want to experience again. I am going to ask you to eat one meal today, preferably breakfast but not more than 300 calories. For the remainder of the day I will ask that you have only fluids. Choose whichever fluids you like with the exception of milk drinks, shakes, smoothies, soda, and alcohol. Be sure to include water. I am basically asking you to fast for one day out of the week and eat as little for breakfast as possible. I am asking you to do this because when you feel the satisfaction from having accomplished this, you will want to do it again. Fasting one day out of the week will make you healthier physically and mentally.

NOTE: *Always check with your doctor first before engaging in any type of fast.*

Option 3:
Self-Control/Discipline-Rooted Diet Plan
(Begin on Day 8 or Day 15)

Finally, I'd like for you to do something that will give you great results in seeing weight loss in your body. I also consider it to be a lifestyle adjustment, which is what this book is all about: creating a healthier lifestyle that you can live with forever. I would like for you to not eat anything past 7:30 PM on a daily basis. I'm well aware that some of you don't get home until after this time. I will ask that you plan accordingly by eating a larger, more fulfilling breakfast and/or lunch or eat before you take that long car, train, or bus ride home. Go sit and have a bite to eat before you head home if your commute will get you home after 7:30 PM. Whatever you need to do, make the adjustment. I highly recommend this diet plan so that you receive the gratification from the results of sticking to this plan.

It is my hope that you will continue the Self-Control-Rooted, Discipline-Rooted, and Self-Control/Discipline-Rooted Diet Plans in your daily living after the forty days. These are small but significant lifestyle changes that will bring extraordinary benefits. My definition of self-control is having control over acting on one's desires. My definition of discipline is to have mastered not acting on one's desires by having practiced self-control. If you possess these, you possess the ability to be successful in never having a stronghold take control over your life—not food, not anything. My definition of stronghold is a wrong mindset that does not honor God in believing that He will help to deliver you from something that is keeping you in bondage.

NOTE: Please remember to bow, or lift, your heads and pray before beginning these diet plans.

GOD'S PLAN
For Total Renewal

(Begin when you are ready for a personal
relationship with God)

Hopefully, you have prayed to God at the beginning of every exercise and have spoken and meditated on His Word at the end of every exercise. I pray that you recognize and acknowledge Him in your forty-day journey. You are truly blessed. It is my prayer that you will want Jesus to be the cornerstone of your life in all things. God is the Author of our lives. There is no one Who knows us better than He. He created us for His purpose, and we should surrender our lives to Him with our complete trust in Him.

God's Plan is that we know Him through having a personal relationship with Him. He has given us the Holy Bible for this instruction. The most important decision you will ever make in your life is the decision to accept God's gift to us, which is salvation through His Son, Jesus Christ. God's Plan is for us to spend life with Him, through Jesus, in this present life and after this life, according to His principles. The minute we accept Jesus Christ, we enter eternal life. You definitely have to wait until you get to Heaven for the home that awaits you there, but God wants to give you a great many awesome things in this present life. Unfortunately, you will never receive them nor experience the relationship with God that He desires with you if you never come to know Jesus. Do you realize that if you pray to God, call Him "Father," talk to Him, want and hope for Him to answer your prayers, that it is God who put His name in your heart? "If God gives such attention to the appearance of wildflowers—most of which are never even seen—don't you think He'll attend to you, take pride in you, do His best for you? What I'm trying to do here is to get you to relax, to not be so preoccupied with *get-*

ting, so you can respond to God's *giving.* People who don't know God and the way He works fuss over these things, but you know both God and how He works" (Matthew 6:30-32 The Message).

I recommend that you do each and every exercise and follow every diet plan in this book on your journey to wellness. If I were to choose the most important plan for you to follow in this book, it would be "God's Plan." "Steep your life in God-reality, God-initiative, God-provisions. Don't worry about missing out. You'll find all your everyday human concerns will be met" (Matthew 6:33 The Message). When you live life according to God's principles, you are truly blessed. God is in every part of your life. As long as you seek Him first in all things, life will be excellent in that you will always be in the presence of the Lord. John 3:16 (The Message) says, "This is how much God loved the world: He gave His Son, His one and only Son. And this is why: so that no one need be destroyed; by believing in Him, anyone can have a whole and lasting life."

Romans 10:8-10 (The Message) states, "So what exactly was Moses saying? The word that saves is right here, as near as the tongue in your mouth, as close as the heart in your chest. It's the word of faith that welcomes God to go to work and set things right for us. This is the core of our preaching. Say the welcoming word to God—'Jesus is my Master'—embracing, body and soul, God's work of doing in us what He did in raising Jesus from the dead. That's it. You're not 'doing' anything; you're simply calling out to God, trusting Him to do it for you. That's salvation. With your whole being you embrace God setting things right, and then you say it, right out loud: 'God has set everything right between Him and me!'"

If you are ready to make Jesus Lord of your life, have your life renewed, and begin your personal relationship with

God, please bow or lift your head and speak with your whole heart this prayer of salvation:

Dear Father, thank You for opening my heart to hear Your call. Thank You for loving me so much that You gave Your only begotten Son to pay the price for my sins by dying on the cross for me. Father, I confess that I am a sinner. I ask for Your forgiveness for my sins. With my whole heart I turn away from my sins. I wholeheartedly believe that Jesus is Lord and surrender my entire life to Him. He is in control. Please fill me with wisdom and understanding of Your Word and help me to follow You in all ways so that I may fulfill Your purpose for my life and always live a life that is pleasing to You. Father, I love You with all my heart, with all my soul, and with all my strength. In Jesus' Name, Amen.

Welcome to the Kingdom! Let the extraordinary life begin. Pray to God for His direction to a good Bible-believing church that honors what Jesus did for you on the cross and provides instruction and community where you can grow.

Day 8

Warm-Up Prayer:

Let us bow, or lift, our heads and pray. You can pray your own prayer, use the one below, or do both.

Dear Father, I sing praise to You forever for turning the mourning of an unhealthy body into the dancing of a healthy body for me. May I not be silent, and with everything that You have made me and allow me to be, for Your purpose, sing the song of gladness that is in my heart. O Lord, my Rock, my Redeemer, I will thank You all the days of my life for removing this stronghold from my life that kept me unhealthy for so long. In Jesus' Name, Amen.

Exercise: Body Twists

Always remember to breathe in and out through your nose. Stand or sit up straight, stretch your arms out shoulder height and slowly twist your upper body to the left, twist your upper body to the front, and then twist your upper body to the right. Repeat this exercise for forty counts. Rest as needed.

NOTE: *This exercise can be performed in a standing or sitting position.*

Cool-Down Scripture (Speak This):

Give instruction to a wise man and he will be yet wiser; teach a righteous man (one upright and in right standing with God) and he will increase in learning. The reverent and worshipful fear of the Lord is the beginning (the chief and choice part) of Wisdom, and the knowledge of the Holy One is insight and understanding. For by me [Wisdom from God] your days shall be multiplied, and the years of your life shall be increased. If you are wise, you are wise for yourself; if you scorn, you alone will bear it and pay the penalty. (Proverbs 9:9-12 AMP)

CHAPTER TWO

Day 9

Warm-Up Prayer:

Let us bow, or lift, our heads and pray. You can pray your own prayer, use the Scripture below, or do both.

ASCRIBE TO the Lord, O sons of the mighty, ascribe to the Lord glory and strength. Give to the Lord the glory due to His name; worship the Lord in the beauty of holiness or in holy array. The voice of the Lord is upon the waters; the God of glory thunders; the Lord is upon many (great) waters. The voice of the Lord is powerful; the voice of the Lord is full of majesty. (Psalm 29:1-4 AMP)

Exercise: Leg Raise

Always remember to breathe in and out through your nose. While lying down, place your hands in a praying hands position and rest them on your abdomen. Raise your legs straight up, while raising your hands at the same time. Then lower them back down together, slowly. Remember to keep your hands in the praying hands position. If you find it easier to raise one leg at a time, do this. Repeat this exercise for forty counts. Remember to rest as needed.

NOTE: This exercise should be performed in a lying position only and may be more easily done with a pillow placed under your backside.

Cool-Down Scripture (Speak This):

Step out of the traffic! Take a long, loving look at me, your High God, above politics, above everything. (Psalm 46:10 The Message)

Day 10

Warm-Up Prayer:

Let us bow, or lift, our heads and pray. You can pray your own prayer, use the one below, or do both.

Dear Father, thank You for wisdom and understanding of Your Word. I love You with a reverent and worshipful fear. Obedience and faith bless me all of the days of my life. In Jesus' Name, Amen.

Exercise: Leg Hugs

Always remember to breathe in and out through your nose. Stand straight; bend your upper body down at the waist, bringing your head towards your knees as much as possible while sliding your hands down your legs; and then grab the backs of your knees. Legs may be bent or straight, whichever is more comfortable for you. Do not worry if you aren't able to bend all the way to your knees. Return to original standing position. This will seem very difficult to do at first but will get easier with practice. Repeat for forty counts. Remember to rest as needed.

NOTE: *This exercise should be performed in a standing position only.*

Cool-Down Scripture (Speak This):

    Lady Wisdom has built and furnished her home; it's supported by seven hewn timbers. The banquet meal is ready to be served: lamb roasted, wine poured out, table set with silver and flowers. Having dismissed her serving maids, Lady Wisdom goes to town, stands in a prominent place, and invites everyone within sound of her voice: "Are you confused about life, don't know what's going on? Come with me, oh come, have dinner with me! I've prepared a wonderful spread—fresh-baked bread, roast lamb, carefully selected wines. Leave your impoverished confusion and live! Walk up the street to a life with meaning."
    If you reason with an arrogant cynic, you'll get slapped in the face; confront bad behavior and get a kick in the shins. So don't waste your time on a scoffer; all you'll get for your pains is abuse. But if you correct those who care about life, that's different—they'll love you for it! Save your breath for the wise—they'll be wiser for it; tell good people what you know—they'll profit from it. Skilled living gets its start in the Fear-of-God, insight into life from knowing a Holy God. It's through me, Lady Wisdom, that your life deepens, and the years of your life ripen. (Proverbs 9:1-11 The Message)

Day 11

Warm-Up Prayer:

Let us bow, or lift, our heads and pray. You can pray your own prayer, use the one below, or do both.

Dear Lord, please give me supernatural motivation and strength to exercise continually, bringing healing to my insides as well as my outsides. Help me to see my inner life changing as well as my outer life. Help me to see all of the beautiful things that You have blessed me with. Search me, oh Lord, and clean my insides so that my outsides emerge anew. In Jesus' Name, Amen.

Exercise: Happy Shoulders

Always remember to breathe in and out through your nose. Shrug your shoulders by moving your shoulders up and down with no help from any other part of your body. Place your hands in a praying position while doing this and repeat for forty counts. Remember to rest as needed.

NOTE: *This exercise can be performed in a standing, sitting, or lying position.*

Cool-Down Scripture (Speak This):

Welcome to the living Stone, the source of life. The workmen took one look and threw it out; God set it in the place of honor. Present yourselves as building stones for the construction of a sanctuary vibrant with life, in which you'll serve as holy priests offering Christ-approved lives up to God. The Scriptures provide precedent: Look! I'm setting a stone in Zion, a cornerstone in the place of honor. Whoever trusts in this stone as a foundation will never have cause to regret it. To you who trust Him, He's a Stone to be proud of, but to those who refuse to trust Him, The stone the workmen threw out is now the chief foundation stone. For the untrusting it's a stone to trip over, a boulder blocking the way. They trip and fall because they refuse to obey, just as predicted. (1 Peter 2:4-8 The Message)

Day 12

Warm-Up Prayer:

Let us bow, or lift, our heads and pray. You can pray your own prayer, use the one below, or do both.

Dear Father, I fret not because of evil men. I will continue to do good, persevere, and be diligently bold and fearless in all of my activities. Lord, my trust is in You. I delight myself in You, dear Father. Thank You for blessing me with the desires of my heart. In Jesus' Name, Amen.

Exercise: Tummy Tuck

Always remember to breathe in and out through your nose. Take a deep breath and then release (do not move your body) while you slowly pull your navel into your stomach as far as you can, hold for a moment, exhale fully, and then relax. Do this exercise at a comfortable pace. Do not perform this exercise quickly. Repeat this for forty counts. Remember to rest as needed.

NOTE: *This exercise can be performed in a standing, sitting, or lying position.*

Cool-Down Scripture (Speak This):

God hates cheating in the marketplace; He loves it when business is aboveboard. The stuck-up fall flat on their faces, but down-to-earth people stand firm. The integrity of the honest keeps them on track; the deviousness of crooks brings them to ruin. A thick bankroll is no help when life falls apart, but a principled life can stand up to the worst. (Proverbs 11:1-4 The Message)

Day 13

Warm-Up Prayer:

Let us bow, or lift, our heads and pray. You can pray your own prayer, use the Scripture below, or do both.

Not for our sake, GOD, no, not for our sake, but for Your name's sake, show Your glory. Do it on account of Your merciful love, do it on account of Your faithful ways. (Psalm 115:1 The Message)

Exercise: Head Moves

Always remember to breathe in and out through your nose. In a sitting position, bend your head down towards your chest and back up, repeating for ten counts; backwards and back up for ten counts; to the right side and back up for ten counts; and finally to the left side and back up for ten counts. The rest of the body should remain still. Remember to rest as needed.

NOTE: *This exercise should be performed in a sitting position only.*

Cool-Down Scripture (Speak This):

So here's what I want you to do, God helping you: Take your everyday, ordinary life—your sleeping, eating, going-to-work, and walking-around life—and place it before God as an offering. Embracing what God does for you is the best thing you can do for Him. (Romans 12:1 The Message)

Day 14

Warm-Up Prayer:

Let us bow, or lift, our heads and pray. You can pray your own prayer, use the one below, or do both.

Dear Father, I love You. For You turned Your ear to my cry for mercy. I will call on You all the days of my life. In Jesus' Name, Amen.

Exercise: One-Legged Stand

Always remember to breathe in and out through your nose. Stand straight and lift your right leg up off the floor towards your front. Leg may be bent or straight, whichever is more comfortable for you. Remain in this position while you count to twenty and then lower your right leg. Next, lift your left leg up off the floor towards your front and remain in this position while you count to twenty. Lower your left leg. Rest as needed.

NOTE: *This exercise should be performed in a standing position only. Please do* ***not*** *use a chair for support in this exercise, unless it is absolutely necessary. This exercise is for achieving better balance.*

Cool-Down Scripture (Speak This):

Good friend, take to heart what I'm telling you; collect my counsels and guard them with your life. Tune your ears to the world of Wisdom; set your heart on a life of Understanding. That's right—if you make Insight your priority, and won't take no for an answer, Searching for it like a prospector panning for gold, like an adventurer on a treasure hunt, Believe me, before you know it Fear-of-God will be yours; you'll have come upon the Knowledge of God. And here's why: God gives out Wisdom free, is plainspoken in Knowledge and Understanding. He's a rich mine of Common Sense for those who live well, a personal bodyguard to the candid and sincere. He keeps His eye on all who live honestly, and pays special attention to His loyally committed ones. So now you can pick out what's true and fair, find all the good trails! Lady Wisdom will be your close friend, and Brother Knowledge your pleasant companion. (Proverbs 2:1-10 The Message)

Day 15

Warm-Up Prayer:

Let us bow, or lift, our heads and pray. You can pray your own prayer, use the one below, or do both.

Dear Father, Your grace is sufficient for me. Your power is made perfect in weakness. I am from You and Your Spirit lives in me. I once was weak and now I am strong. Thank You for giving me the wisdom to recognize and acknowledge the power that I've been given. I run boldly to challenges. Victory is mine. In Jesus' Name, Amen.

Exercise: Flat-out Stretching

Always remember to breathe in and out through your nose. Lie on your stomach. Place your hands on your waist and lift both legs up, bending at the knees and bringing them as close to your backside as possible, then lower both legs down slowly. Repeat this for forty counts. Remember to rest as needed.

NOTE*: This exercise should be performed in a lying position only.*

Cool-Down Scripture (Speak This):

Don't lie to one another. You're done with that old life. It's like a filthy set of ill-fitting clothes you've stripped off and put in the fire. Now you're dressed in a new wardrobe. Every item of your new way of life is custom-made by the Creator, with His label on it. (Colossians 3:9-10 The Message)

***REMINDER:** Have you chosen one or more of the diet plans? Have you chosen God's Plan?*

Day 16

Warm-Up Prayer:

Let us bow, or lift, our heads and pray. You can pray your own prayer, use the one below, or do both.

Our Father Who art in Heaven, I press forward to the best that my body can be by using my body, soul, and spirit, knowing that all good gifts come from the Lord. My body is the temple. We have to reclaim our bodies. We treat our bodies just like they are of the world and not just in the world. We put all types of foods in our bodies because they taste good. If you feel good in health, you will look good. Dear Father, thank You for helping me to feel good and look good. In Jesus' Name, Amen.

Exercise: Toe Stretch

Always remember to breathe in and out through your nose. On both feet, move your toes by pointing them upwards and downwards, to the left and to the right. Repeat this for forty counts. Remember to rest as needed.

NOTE: This exercise can be performed in a standing, sitting, or lying position.

Cool-Down Scripture (Speak This):

Gracious speech is like clover honey—good taste to the soul, quick energy for the body. (Proverbs 16:24 The Message)

CHAPTER THREE

Day 17

Warm-Up Prayer:

Let us bow, or lift, our heads and pray. You can pray your own prayer, use the one below, or do both.

Dear Father, thank You for You, Jesus, and the Holy Spirit. Thank You for Your renewed mercy each and every morning and Your grace. Thank You for enriching me in every way with all kinds of speech, knowledge, and wisdom to discern what is good. Thank You for instilling in me a passion to pursue what is true, always in unbroken fellowship and faith. In Jesus' Name, Amen.

Exercise: Elbow Stretch

Always remember to breathe in and out through your nose. Cross your legs in an "X" position where one is behind the other and your feet are flat on the floor. Place your hands behind your head and lock fingers. Bring your elbows together as far as you can where they almost touch, then stretch them back out and bring them in again. Repeat this for forty counts. Remember to rest as needed.

NOTE: This exercise should be performed in a sitting position only.

Cool-Down Scripture (Speak This):

Every time I think of you—and I think of you often!—I thank God for your lives of free and open access to God, given by Jesus. There's no end to what has happened in you—it's beyond speech, beyond knowledge. The evidence of Christ has been clearly verified in your lives. Just think— you don't need a thing, you've got it all! All God's gifts are right in front of you as you wait expectantly for our Master Jesus to arrive on the scene for the Finale. And not only that, but God Himself is right alongside to keep you steady and on track until things are all wrapped up by Jesus. God, Who got you started in this spiritual adventure, shares with us the life of His Son and our Master Jesus. He will never give up on you. Never forget that. (1 Corinthians 1:4-9 The Message)

Day 18

Warm-Up Prayer:

Let us bow, or lift, our heads and pray. You can pray your own prayer, use the Scripture below, or do both.

When I walk into the thick of trouble, keep me alive in the angry turmoil. With one hand strike my foes, With Your other hand save me. Finish what You started in me, GOD. Your love is eternal—don't quit on me now. (Psalm 138:7-8 The Message)

Exercise: Almost Sitting

Always remember to breathe in and out through your nose. Stand in front of a chair, with your back to its seat. Holding onto the armrest, if available, bend as if you are going to sit down, only do not let your backside touch the chair. Then slowly rise up and repeat this for forty counts. Remember to rest as needed. This is a good exercise for strengthening your legs and shaping your backside.

NOTE: This exercise should be performed in a standing position only and requires the use of a chair.

Cool-Down Scripture (Speak This):

Well-spoken words bring satisfaction; well-done work has its own reward. (Proverbs 12:14 The Message)

Day 19

Warm-Up Prayer:

Let us bow, or lift, our heads and pray. You can pray your own prayer, use the one below, or do both.

Dear Father, please continue to give me the strength, energy, and focus to do the following exercise in order that my arms and legs become new. Thank You for strengthening my arms and getting rid of the flappers as well as my legs, the clappers. A little humor, Father, but You know what I mean. Thank You for giving me newly shaped arms and legs. In Jesus' Name, Amen.

Exercise: Stretch and Lift

Always remember to breathe in and out through your nose. Stand straight, stretch your right arm out in front of you, while simultaneously stretching your right leg out in front as well, lifting your leg upwards towards your hand. Leg may be bent or straight, whichever is more comfortable for you. Then lower your right arm and right leg and repeat this for ten counts. Stretch your left arm out in front of you, while simultaneously stretching your left leg out in front as well, lifting your leg upwards towards your hand. Then lower your left arm and left leg and repeat this for ten counts.

Repeat this exercise by alternately stretching your right arm and right leg and then your left arm and left leg out to the side for ten counts each. Remember to rest as needed. This is a good exercise for strengthening your legs and shaping your backside.

NOTE: *This exercise should be performed in a standing position only and may be more easily done using a chair for support.*

Cool-Down Scripture (Speak This):

GOD is my strength, GOD is my song, and, yes! GOD is my salvation. *This* is the kind of God I have and I'm telling the world! *This* is the God of my father—I'm spreading the news far and wide! (Exodus 15:2 The Message)

Day 20

Warm-Up Prayer:

Let us bow, or lift, our heads and pray. You can pray your own prayer, use the one below, or do both.

Dear Father, I am halfway through the exercises that are jumpstarting me to a new and healthier life. Thank You for filling my heart with doing the right things for me. In Jesus' Name, Amen.

Exercise: Moving Still

Always remember to breathe in and out through your nose. Stand straight and start moving your legs in a running motion; run in place slowly, repeating this for ten counts. Slowly change to a faster but comfortable pace for ten counts. Now move to a very fast pace for ten counts. Then slow down to a very slow speed for ten counts. Remember to rest as needed.

NOTE: *This exercise should be performed in a standing position only.*

Cool-Down Scripture (Speak This):

That is what happened in baptism. When we went under the water, we left the old country of sin behind; when we came up out of the water, we entered into the new country of grace—a new life in a new land! That's what baptism into the life of Jesus means. When we are lowered into the water, it is like the burial of Jesus; when we are raised up out of the water, it is like the resurrection of Jesus. Each of us is raised into a light-filled world by our Father so that we can see where we're going in our new grace-sovereign country. (Romans 6:3-5 The Message)

Day 21

Warm-Up Prayer:

Let us bow, or lift, our heads and pray. You can pray your own prayer, use the one below, or do both.

Dear Father, thank You for waking me up this morning. Thank You for Your renewed mercy and Your grace. Thank You for giving me the strength, diligence, and endurance to continue my exercise regimen. In Jesus' Name, Amen.

Exercise: Swimming on Dry Land

Always remember to breathe in and out through your nose. Lie down on your stomach and place your hands out in front of you. Head face down, stretch your legs out behind you and lift your right leg while you simultaneously lift your left arm. Then lower your right leg and left arm as you lift your left leg and right arm, like you're swimming. Don't let your legs touch the floor or bed. Repeat this for forty counts. Remember to rest as needed.

NOTE: *This exercise should be performed in a lying position only.*

Cool-Down Prayer (Speak This):

Dear Father, thank You for the exercises You have just strengthened me to do. My body is getting healthier and reshaping to be a better vessel in which You dwell. Thank You for teaching me that I can do all things through You Who strengthens me. In Jesus' Name, Amen.

Day 22

Warm-Up Prayer:

Let us bow, or lift, our heads and pray. You can pray your own prayer, use the one below, or do both.

Dear Father, thank You for guiding me into a healthier life physically, mentally, and spiritually. I pray that this is also reflected in my relationships as well. In Jesus' Name, Amen.

Exercise: Uplifting Praise

Always remember to breathe in and out through your nose. Slowly bring your arms out to your sides and lift them up all the way to where your hands touch over your head, in a praying position. Slowly bring them back down to your sides. Repeat this for forty counts. Remember to rest as needed.

NOTE: *This exercise can be performed in a standing, sitting, or lying position.*

Cool-Down Scripture (Speak This):

If you do well, won't you be accepted? And if you don't do well, sin is lying in wait for you, ready to pounce; it's out to get you, you've got to master it. (Genesis 4:7 The Message)

Day 23

Warm-Up Prayer:

Let us bow, or lift, our heads and pray. You can pray your own prayer, use the one below, or do both.

Father, thank You for desiring me as Your child, thank You for teaching me how to exercise and that the exercise does not have to be strenuous but consistent. In Jesus' Name, Amen.

Exercise: Thigh Togetherness

Always remember to breathe in and out through your nose. Place your feet firmly on the floor where they are together and touching. Bring your thighs inwards where your knees touch. Remember to keep your feet in the same position and not move. Hold to the count of forty. Remember to rest as needed. This is a good exercise for strengthening your legs and shaping your backside.

NOTE: *This exercise should be performed in a sitting position only.*

Cool-Down Scripture (Speak This):

They sang antiphonally praise and thanksgiving to God: Yes! God is good! Oh yes—He'll never quit loving Israel! All the people boomed out hurrahs, praising God as the foundation of The Temple of God was laid. (Ezra 3:11 The Message)

Day 24

Warm-Up Prayer:

Let us bow, or lift, our heads and pray. You can pray your own prayer, use the one below, or do both.

Dear Father, thank You for being with me through the day. Thank You for giving me the activity of my limbs. In Jesus' Name, Amen.

Exercise: Arm Lift

Always remember to breathe in and out through your nose. Place your right hand on your left elbow, and place your left hand on your right elbow. With your arms in this position, slowly lift them up over your head as far as you can go without straining and then lower them back down slowly. Repeat this for forty counts. Remember to rest as needed.

NOTE: *This exercise can be performed in a standing, sitting, or lying position.*

Cool-Down Scripture (Speak This):

You who sit down in the High God's presence, spend the night in Shaddai's shadow, Say this: "GOD, You're my refuge. I trust in You and I'm safe!" (Psalm 91:1-2 The Message)

CHAPTER FOUR

Day 25

Warm-Up Prayer:

Let us bow, or lift, our heads and pray. You can pray your own prayer, use the one below, or do both.

Father, thank You for all that You are doing for my body. Thank You for caring and instilling in me the desire to care as well. Thank You for teaching me wisdom, understanding, and diligence. In Jesus' Name, Amen.

Exercise: Body Stretching

Always remember to breathe in and out through your nose. Lie down on your back and stretch out into a straight line with your arms overhead and your legs flat on the floor. Raise your upper body slightly towards your knees as you bend your knees in towards you and then release while stretching your legs and arms back down in a straight line. Try not to let your legs or arms touch the floor or bed while stretching. Repeat this for forty counts. Remember to rest as needed.

NOTE: This exercise should be performed in a lying position only and may be more easily done with a pillow placed under your backside.

Cool-Down Scripture (Speak This):

God gave Solomon wisdom—the deepest of understanding and the largest of hearts. There was nothing beyond him, nothing he couldn't handle. (1 Kings 4:29 The Message)

Day 26

Warm-Up Prayer:

Let us bow, or lift, our heads and pray. You can pray your own prayer, use the one below, or do both.

Father, please help me to do these exercises this morning. Please help me to want to do these exercises this morning, Father. Please send to me Your supernatural power, strength, focus, diligence, and, most of all, energy so I can do these exercises with zeal. In Jesus' Name, Amen.

Exercise: Eye Strengthening

Always remember to breathe in and out through your nose. Keep your head still and look to the right, look to the left, look up, and then look down. Repeat this for twenty counts. Now, without moving your head, draw a circle with your eyes. Repeat this for twenty counts. This is a good eye exercise for someone who has been reading all day or has been working on the computer. You can do this exercise at any speed that you like; however, it is most comfortable to move at a slow to moderate pace. Remember to rest as needed.

NOTE: This exercise can be performed in a standing, sitting, or lying position.

Cool-Down Scripture (Speak This):

The people who walked in darkness have seen a great light. For those who lived in a land of deep shadows—light! sunbursts of light! You repopulated the nation, You expanded its joy. Oh, they're so glad in Your presence! Festival joy! The joy of a great celebration, sharing rich gifts and warm greetings. The abuse of oppressors and cruelty of tyrants—all their whips and cudgels and curses—Is gone, done away with, a deliverance as surprising and sudden as Gideon's old victory over Midian. (Isaiah 9:2-4 The Message)

Day 27

Warm-Up Prayer:

Let us bow, or lift, our heads and pray. You can pray your own prayer, use the one below, or do both.

Dear Father, thank You for a peaceful heart; giving life to my body. May the meditation of my heart and the words of my mouth never be filled with envy. In Jesus' Name, Amen.

Exercise: Thigh Massage

Always remember to breathe in and out through your nose. Lying on your back, raise your right leg up. Take both hands and place it on your right thigh, while gently pressing down on the thigh in a massaging motion up and down. Slowly lower your leg down and then repeat this for twenty counts. Then raise your left leg up. Take both hands and place it on your left thigh, while gently pressing down on the thigh in a massaging motion up and down. Slowly lower your leg down and then repeat this for twenty counts. Remember to rest as needed.

NOTE*: This exercise should be performed in a lying position only.*

Cool-Down Scripture (Speak This):

A sound mind makes for a robust body, but runaway emotions corrode the bones. (Proverbs 14:30 The Message)

Day 28

Warm-Up Prayer:

Let us bow, or lift, our heads and pray. You can pray your own prayer, use the Scripture below, or do both.

O my soul, bless God. From head to toe, I'll bless His holy name! O my soul, bless God, don't forget a single blessing! He forgives your sins—every one. He heals your diseases—every one. He redeems you from hell—saves your life! He crowns you with love and mercy—a paradise crown. He wraps you in goodness—beauty eternal. He renews your youth—you're always young in His presence. God makes everything come out right; He puts victims back on their feet. (Psalm 103:1-6 The Message)

Exercise: Piano Move

Always remember to breathe in and out through your nose. Slowly raise your arms in the air as high as they will go while simultaneously moving your fingers in a piano-playing motion. Slowly let your arms down, keep playing the piano. Repeat this for forty counts. This is an arm and finger strengthening exercise. Remember to rest as needed.

NOTE: *This exercise can be performed in a standing, sitting, or lying position.*

Cool-Down Scripture (Speak This):

Come, let's shout praises to GOD, raise the roof for the Rock who saved us! Let's march into His presence singing praises, lifting the rafters with our hymns! And why? Because GOD is the best, High King over all the gods. In one hand He holds deep caves and caverns, in the other hand grasps the high mountains. He made Ocean—He owns it! His hands sculpted Earth! So come, let us worship: bow before Him, on your knees before God, who made us! (Psalm 95:1-6 The Message)

Day 29

Warm-Up Prayer:

Let us bow, or lift, our heads and pray. You can pray your own prayer, use the Scripture below, or do both.

Light, space, zest— that's GOD! So, with Him on my side I'm fearless, afraid of no one and nothing. (Psalm 27:1 The Message)

Exercise: Graceful Arms

Always remember to breathe in and out through your nose. Slowly bring your arms out in front of you while opening and closing your hands, stretch them out to the side, then slowly bring them back in. Remember to keep opening and closing your hands in this exercise. This may seem easy, but it is a powerful exercise for the shoulders, arms, hands, and fingers. Repeat this for forty counts. Rest as needed.

NOTE: This exercise can be performed in a standing, sitting, or lying position.

Cool-Down Scripture (Speak This):

Sing GOD a brand-new song! Earth and everyone in it, sing! Sing to God—worship GOD! Shout the news of His victory from sea to sea, Take the news of His glory to the lost, News of His wonders to one and all! For GOD is great, and worth a thousand Hallelujahs. His terrible beauty makes the gods look cheap; Pagan gods are mere tatters and rags. GOD made the Heavens—Royal splendor radiates from Him, A powerful beauty sets Him apart. (Psalm 96:1-6 The Message)

Day 30

Warm-Up Prayer:

Let us bow, or lift, our heads and pray. You can pray your own prayer, use the one below, or do both.

Dear Father, please help me to carefully watch and guard the words that come out of my mouth and the thoughts that are in my heart so that both are always pleasing in Your sight. In Jesus' Name, Amen.

Exercise: Leg Strengthening

Always remember to breathe in and out through your nose. Get into a chair, any type of chair that is comfortable to you. Raise your legs up together no higher than your waist or as far as they will go, then slowly bring them back down. Leg movement hinges at the knees, and upper legs should remain on the seat. Repeat this for forty counts. Remember to rest as needed.

NOTE: *This exercise should be performed in a sitting position only.*

Cool-Down Scripture (Speak This):

Keep vigilant watch over your heart; that's where life starts. Don't talk out of both sides of your mouth; avoid careless banter, white lies, and gossip. (Proverbs 4:23-24 The Message)

Day 31

Warm-Up Prayer:

Let us bow, or lift, our heads and pray. You can pray your own prayer, use the one below, or do both.

Dear Father, as I begin Day 31 of my exercise regimen, please strengthen me, keep me focused, and guide me into having the exact body that You and I both desire for me. Please help me to enjoy the exercises that I do and to incorporate them into my daily living beyond Day 40. In Jesus' Name, Amen.

Exercise: Heel/Toe

Always remember to breathe in and out through your nose. While sitting, take your right foot and slightly lift it off the floor while pointing your toes upwards and then downwards. Try not to let your foot touch the floor. Repeat this for twenty counts. Then take your left foot and slightly lift it off the floor while pointing your toes upwards and then downwards. Try not to let your foot touch the floor. Repeat this for twenty counts. Remember to rest as needed.

NOTE: *This exercise should be performed in a sitting position only.*

Cool-Down Scripture (Speak This):

Love God, your God, with your whole heart: love Him with all that's in you, love Him with all you've got! (Deuteronomy 6:5 The Message)

Day 32

Warm-Up Prayer:

Let us bow, or lift, our heads and pray. You can pray your own prayer, use the one below, or do both.

Dear Father, as I begin Day 32 of my exercise regimen I pray that my body is forming into greatness that will remain for the rest of my life. I pray that it will never be in me to eat the wrong things that bring no good to my body. In Jesus' Name, Amen.

Exercise: Nostril Opening

Always remember to breathe in and out through your nose. Slowly open and close your nostrils as you take deep breaths in and out. Do not use anything but your breath and nostril muscles to open and close them. Repeat this for forty counts. Remember to rest as needed.

NOTE: *This exercise can be performed in a standing, sitting, or lying position and is good for reducing stress.*

Cool-Down Scripture (Speak This):

Know this: GOD, your God, is God indeed, a God you can depend upon. He keeps His covenant of loyal love with those who love Him and observe His commandments for a thousand generations. (Deuteronomy 7:9 The Message)

CHAPTER FIVE

Day 33

Warm-Up Prayer:

Let us bow, or lift, our heads and pray. You can pray your own prayer, use the one below, or do both.

Dear Father, as I lean on You, please help me to keep my balance. I can do all things through Christ, Who strengthens me. In Jesus' Name, Amen.

Exercise: Drawing a Moon

Sit in a chair or on the bed for this exercise. Always remember to breathe in and out through your nose. Lift your right leg off the floor and move it in a circular motion inward, repeating for ten counts and then outward for ten counts. Leg may be bent or straight, whichever is more comfortable for you. Lower your right leg, and then lift your left leg off the floor and move it in a circular motion inward for ten counts and outward for ten counts. Lower your left leg. Remember to rest as needed.

NOTE: *This exercise should be performed in a sitting position only.*

Cool-Down Scripture (Speak This):

Trust God from the bottom of your heart; don't try to figure out everything on your own. Listen for God's voice in everything you do, everywhere you go; He's the One who will keep you on track. (Proverbs 3:5-6 The Message)

Day 34

Warm-Up Prayer:

Let us bow, or lift, our heads and pray. You can pray your own prayer, use the one below, or do both.

Dear Father, thank You from the depths of my heart for giving me supernatural strength, power, motivation, and diligence to get to this point where I have consistently done thirty-three days of exercise. Thank You for the remolding of my outsides. May both my insides and my outsides be pleasing in Your eyes. In Jesus' Name, Amen.

Exercise: Upper Body Stretch

Always remember to breathe in and out through your nose. Lie down on your back and stretch out into a straight line with your arms overhead and your legs flat on the floor or bed. Clasp your fingers behind your head and raise your upper body as far as it will go, without totally sitting all of the way up, and then slowly lie back down. Be careful not to pull on the neck but to use your abdominal muscles to raise your upper body. Repeat this exercise for forty counts. Remember to rest as needed.

NOTE: This exercise should be performed in a lying position only and may be more easily done with a pillow placed under your backside.

Cool-Down Scripture (Speak This):

Clear lots of ground for your tents! Make your tents large. Spread out! Think big! Use plenty of rope, drive the tent pegs deep. (Isaiah 54:2 The Message)

Day 35

Warm-Up Prayer:

Let us bow, or lift, our heads and pray. You can pray your own prayer, use the one below, or do both.

Dear Father, I can hardly believe the results I am seeing. Thank You for keeping me focused and motivated and for guiding me to wellness. Thank You for where You've brought me. May I always follow You. In Jesus' Name, Amen.

Exercise: Bend, Slide, Squat

Always remember to breathe in and out through your nose. Slowly bend forward while sliding your hands down your legs and grasping both ankles. Hold your ankles while slightly bending your knees to a squatting position, hold for a second then unbend your knees while still touching your ankles, slide your hands back up your legs and thighs and come to a standing position. Repeat this exercise for forty counts. Remember to rest as needed. This is a good exercise for the backside.

NOTE: *This exercise should be performed in a standing position only.*

Cool-Down Scripture (Speak This):

He shows me how to fight; I can bend a bronze bow! (2 Samuel 22:35 The Message)

Day 36

Warm-Up Prayer:

Let us bow, or lift, our heads and pray. You can pray your own prayer, use the one below, or do both.

Dear Father, thank You for guiding me to a healthier way of living. You equip me to do all things, in Your Will. If You're not a part of it, I want no part in it. Thank You for being my Rock and my Redeemer. In Jesus' Name, Amen.

Exercise: Side Kick

Always remember to breathe in and out through your nose. Slightly lean your upper body to the left and kick your right leg out to the side and up as high as it will go (but do not worry if it is not very far out or up). Leg may be bent or straight, whichever is more comfortable for you. Then lower your leg down slowly and place your foot on the floor while bringing your body into a straight position. Repeat this for twenty counts. Then do the exercise leaning your upper body to the right and using the left leg for twenty counts. Remember to rest as needed.

NOTE: This exercise should be performed in a standing position only.

Cool-Down Scripture (Speak This):

Point me down Your highway, God; direct me along a well-lighted street; show my enemies whose side You're on. (Psalm 27:11 The Message)

Day 37

Warm-Up Prayer:

Let us bow, or lift, our heads and pray. You can pray your own prayer, use the one below, or do both.

Dear Father, thank You for teaching me that I can do all things through Christ, Who strengthens me to do what is in Your Will for me to do. It was Your Will that I become healthy and I thank You and praise Your Holy Name for what You have done for me inside and out. In Jesus' Name, Amen.

Exercise: Bowing Down

Always remember to breathe in and out through your nose. Stand straight with your legs together. Bend over forward to the level of your waist with your arms stretched out to the sides. Hold this position for a couple of seconds, slowly stand up straight, and repeat for forty counts. Remember to rest as needed.

NOTE: *This exercise should be performed in a standing position only.*

Cool-Down Scripture (Speak This):

And also carefully guard yourselves so that you don't look up into the skies and see the sun and moon and stars, all the constellations of the skies, and be seduced into worshiping and serving them. God set them out for everybody's benefit, everywhere. (Deuteronomy 4:19 The Message)

Day 38

Warm-Up Prayer:

Let us bow, or lift, our heads and pray. You can pray your own prayer, use the one below, or do both.

My Father, how awesome You are. Glorious is Thy Name and Thy Character. Thank You for Your Hand and Your Face in this journey of possessing excellent health that we have begun. In Jesus' Name, Amen.

Exercise: Standing Firm

Always remember to breathe in and out through your nose. Stand straight and place your hands on your waist. Lunge forward with your right leg and then come back up to the standing position. Lunge forward with your left leg and then come back up to the standing position. Do this for forty counts. Remember to rest as needed.

NOTE: *This exercise should be performed in a standing position only.*

Cool-Down Scripture (Speak This):

Keep your eyes open, hold tight to your convictions, give it all you've got, be resolute, and love without stopping. (1 Corinthians 16:13-14 The Message)

Day 39

Warm-Up Prayer:

Let us bow, or lift, our heads and pray. You can pray your own prayer, use the one below, or do both.

Father, I can do all things through Christ, Who strengthens me to do the things that He wants me to do. Thank You for healing me from the inside out. In Jesus' Name, Amen.

Exercise: Shake It Off

Always remember to breathe in and out through your nose. Open and close both hands, repeating for ten counts. Move both hands around and around for ten counts. Shake both hands in a waving position (fingers pointing up) for ten counts. Shake both hands in a waving position (fingers pointing down) for ten counts. Remember to rest as needed. This exercise is good for those who work with their hands a lot.

NOTE: This exercise can be performed in a standing, sitting, or lying position.

Cool-Down Scripture (Speak This):

Then [God] picked us up and set us down in highest Heaven in company with Jesus, our Messiah. (Ephesians 2:6 The Message)

The 40-Count Plan

Day 40

Warm-Up Prayer:

Let us bow, or lift, our heads and pray. You can pray your own prayer, use the one below, or do both.

Father, You know my heart. You see me inside and out. How do I begin to thank You for what You have begun in me? I will thank You by continuing this process over and over until You and I are both satisfied with my progress. Thank You for igniting the fire in me to reach Day 40. We have broken the stronghold that was on me and kept me in bondage to the flesh. Thank You for helping to release this stronghold with each day of diligent exercising. Thank You for helping me to reach Day 40 in Your exercise program of choice for me, Father. Thank You for blessing me with The 40-Count Plan. In Jesus' Name, Amen.

Exercise: Defining Muscle

Always remember to breathe in and out through your nose. Place your arms down by your sides; tighten your fists, arms, and shoulder muscles; and then bend your elbows and bring both arms up, fists almost touching your shoulders, as if doing a curl. Imagine weights in each hand. Bring both arms down slowly while holding the tightness in your muscles. Repeat this for forty counts. Try to raise and lower only your arms and not move your shoulders in this exercise. Remember to rest as needed.

NOTE: This exercise can be done while standing, sitting, or lying down.

Cool-Down Scripture (Speak This):

But Moses said, Those aren't songs of victory, And those aren't songs of defeat, I hear songs of people throwing a party. (Exodus 32:18 The Message)

Conclusion

No matter how old you are, as long as you are alive, have faith, and persevere in seeing your dreams become reality, you can do whatever you strive for in life and receive God's blessing on it if you have made Him a part of your life. I had an idea to create an exercise video back in 1976. I believe that it was God's desire that I be the very first person to put out an exercise video, but the seed remained only a seed during that time. Recently, God and I decided to water and grow the seed and give it life by first producing a wellness book and then later having that publication available on video and audiobook. It just goes to show you that when God plants a seed, He will patiently wait on you to step out in faith and water it and help to make it grow, and He will bless it even if it is thirty-five years later, if it is in His Will to do so.

Some of the exercises in this book were thought of long ago, but it wasn't until I was in Alabama taking care of my mother that I began to think of all of the exercises that could be done if you are confined to the bed and how even the least strenuous of exercises are beneficial. Unless you have absolutely no mobility, there is always some type of exercise you can do, even if it is just moving your fingers backwards and forwards and side to side. It was my mother who said to me that trying beats failure. She is correct. Our excuses and need for instant gratification are what keep us from wellness. I know people who have been more successful at being on diets than at losing weight. They started out being overweight and ended up obese because they never stuck with their diet plans. I hope that by the time you get to this page of the book you will have taken full advantage of all of the daily exercises, as well as the unique diet plans, and the plan for total renewal and that you will have overcome the stronghold of excuses. This exercise book is not designed to be like any other. It is intended that when you complete the forty-day plan, you will be physically, mentally, and spiritually healthier and will continue to use this plan in conquering your wellness goals.

This is how much God loved the world: He gave His Son, His one and only Son. And this is why: so that no one need be destroyed; by believing in Him, anyone can have a whole and lasting life. God didn't go to all the trouble of sending His Son merely to point an accusing finger, telling the world how bad it was. He came to help, to put the world right again. Anyone who trusts in Him is acquitted; anyone who refuses to trust Him has long since been under the death sentence without knowing it. And why? Because of that person's failure to believe in the one-of-a-kind Son of God when introduced to Him. (John 3:16-18 The Message)

Appendix

Name: _____

Personal Daily Wellness Plan

40-COUNT PLAN EXERCISES	MY FAVORITE EXERCISES (√)		COUNT/ MINUTES
CHAPTER ONE			
Day 1: Face Stretch			
Day 2: The Stand			
Day 3: Knee Bend			
Day 4: Hand Tightening			
Day 5: Open Wide			
Day 6: With Open Arms			
Day 7: Hugging Yourself			
Day 8: Body Twists			
CHAPTER TWO			
Day 9: Leg Raise			
Day 10: Leg Hugs			
Day 11: Happy Shoulders			
Day 12: Tummy Tuck			
Day 13: Head Moves			
Day 14: One-Legged Stand			
Day 15: Flat-out Stretching			
Day 16: Toe Stretch			
CHAPTER THREE			
Day 17: Elbow Stretch			
Day 18: Almost Sitting			
Day 19: Stretch and Lift			
Day 20: Moving Still			
Day 21: Swimming on Dry Land			
Day 22: Uplifting Praise			
Day 23: Thigh Togetherness			
Day 24: Arm Lift			
CHAPTER FOUR			
Day 25: Body Stretching			
Day 26: Eye Strengthening			
Day 27: Thigh Massage			
Day 28: Piano Move			
Day 29: Graceful Arms			
Day 30: Leg Strengthening			
Day 31: Heel/Toe			
Day 32: Nostril Opening			
CHAPTER FIVE			
Day 33: Drawing a Moon			
Day 34: Upper Body Stretch			
Day 35: Bend, Slide, Squat			
Day 36: Side Kick			
Day 37: Bowing Down			
Day 38: Standing Firm			
Day 39: Shake it Off			
Day 40: Defining Muscle			
	TOTAL MY FAVORITE EXERCISES		**TOTAL COUNT/ MINUTES**

NOTE: **Repeat** The 40-Count Plan *or choose your favorite exercises and include them in your personal daily wellness plan by count or by minutes.*

About The Authors

Pinkie A. Holmes currently resides with her husband in Virginia and is the mother of four daughters and one son. She shows love to everyone that she meets and believes that love is the answer to all of our problems. Never has there been a more dedicated Christian, devoted to spreading the Word of God, living a life approved by Him, helping others, and bringing more souls to Christ. Pinkie is a recent retiree from the brokerage industry and enjoys evangelism and helping others in every way possible. She is also a loving and trusted daughter, sister, grandmother, and aunt. You can visit her on the web through Facebook, and at pinkieholmes@yahoo.com.

Debra La Chelle Dupree currently resides in New York. She is the author of *God's Fragrance: The Fragrance of Life*. She is the mother of a son, who is a devoted educator. Debra is a business professional who has worked in the corporate world in various industries, including advertising, entertainment, oil and gas, finance, insurance, healthcare, and legal. She enjoys writing and interior decorating and is also a loving and trusted daughter, granddaughter, sister, and aunt. You can visit her on the web through Facebook, Twitter, http://debralachelledupree.blogspot.com, and at debradupree@optonline.net.

CPSIA information can be obtained at www.ICGtesting.com
Printed in the USA
BVOW011200050112

279827BV00003B/1/P

9 781600 344732